VEGAN DIET

A manual guidebook on dietary plan for vegeterians

Dr Rowan Theo

Table of Contents

CHAPTER ONE

The Vegan Diet — A Complete Guide for Beginners

Increasingly greater human beings have determined to head vegan for ethical, environmental or fitness reasons.

When performed proper, any such eating regimen may also bring about numerous fitness blessings, consisting of a trimmer waistline and advanced blood sugar manage.

Nevertheless, a eating regimen primarily based totally solely on plant ingredients may also, in a few cases, growth the chance of nutrient deficiencies.

This article is an in depth beginner's manual to the vegan eating regimen. It goals to cowl the whole thing you want to know, so that you can observe a vegan eating regimen the proper manner.

What Is the Vegan Diet?

Veganism is described as a manner of dwelling that tries to exclude all styles of animal exploitation and cruelty, whether or not for meals, garb or every other purpose.

For those reasons, the vegan eating regimen is without all animal merchandise, consisting of meat, eggs and dairy.

People pick to observe a vegan eating regimen for numerous reasons.

These typically variety from ethics to environmental concerns, however they also can stem from a preference to enhance fitness.

BOTTOM LINE:

A vegan eating regimen excludes all animal merchandise. Many human beings pick to consume this manner for ethical, environmental or fitness reasons.

Different Types of Vegan Diets

There are unique types of vegan diets. The maximum common encompass:

• Whole-meals vegan eating regimen: A eating regimen primarily based totally on a extensive sort of entire plant ingredients including fruits, veggies, entire grains, legumes, nuts and seeds.

• Raw-meals vegan eating regimen: A vegan eating regimen primarily based totally on uncooked fruits, veggies, nuts, seeds or plant ingredients cooked at temperatures under 118°F.

• The thrive eating regimen: The thrive eating regimen is a uncooked-meals vegan eating regimen. Followers consume plant-primarily based totally, entire ingredients which might be uncooked or minimally cooked at low temperatures.

• Junk-meals vegan eating regimen: A vegan eating regimen missing in entire plant ingredients that is based closely on mock meats and cheeses, fries, vegan cakes and different closely processed vegan ingredients.

Although numerous versions of the vegan eating regimen exist, maximum medical studies not often differentiates among unique kinds of vegan diets.

Therefore, the records supplied in this text pertains to vegan diets as a entire.

BOTTOM LINE:

There are numerous methods to observe a vegan eating regimen, however medical studies not often differentiates among the unique types.

Vegan Diets Can Help You Lose Weight

Vegans have a tendency to be thinner and feature a decrease frame mass index (BMI) than non-vegans.

This may provide an explanation for why more and more human beings flip to vegan diets as a manner to lose extra weight.

Part of the weight-associated blessings vegans enjoy can be defined with the aid of using elements apart from eating regimen. These may also encompass more healthy way of life choices, including bodily activity, and different fitness-associated behaviors.

However, numerous randomized managed research, which manage for those outside elements, file that vegan diets are greater powerful for weight reduction than the diets they may be as compared to.

Interestingly, the weight reduction benefit persists even if entire-meals-primarily based totally diets are used as manage diets.

What's greater, researchers normally file that contributors on vegan diets lose greater weight than the ones following calorie-confined diets, even if they're allowed to consume till they experience full .

The herbal tendency to consume fewer calorieson a vegan eating regimen can be resulting from a better nutritional fiber consumption, which could make you experience fuller.

BOTTOM LINE:

Vegan diets appear very powerful at assisting human beings obviously lessen the quantity of energy they consume, ensuing in weight reduction.

CHAPTER TWO

Vegan Diets, Blood Sugar and Type 2 Diabetes

Adopting a vegan eating regimen may also assist hold your blood sugar in take a look at and kind 2 diabetes at bay.

Several research display that vegans advantage from decrease blood sugar ranges, better insulin sensitivity and as much as a 78% decrease chance of growing kind 2 diabetes than non-vegans.

In addition, vegan diets reportedly decrease blood sugar ranges in diabetics as much as 2.four instances greater than diets .

Part of the benefit might be defined with the aid of using the better fiber consumption, which may also blunt the blood sugar response. A vegan eating regimen's weight reduction outcomes may also in addition make contributions to its capacity to decrease blood sugar ranges.

BOTTOM LINE:

Vegan diets appear specially powerful at enhancing markers of blood sugar manage. They may additionally decrease the chance of growing kind 2 diabetes.

Vegan Diets and Heart Health

A vegan eating regimen may also assist hold your coronary heart healthy.

Observational research file vegans may also have as much as a 75% decrease chance of growing excessive blood stress and 42% decrease chance of death from coronary heart disorder.

Randomized managed research — the gold general in studies — upload to the proof.

Several file that vegan diets are lots greater powerful at decreasing blood sugar, LDL and overall cholesterol than diets they may be as compared to.

These outcomes might be particularly useful considering that decreasing blood stress, ldl cholesterol and blood sugar may also lessen coronary heart disorder chance with the aid of using as much as 46%.

BOTTOM LINE:

Vegan diets may also enhance coronary heart fitness. However, greater super research are wished earlier than sturdy conclusions may be drawn.

Other Health Benefits of Vegan Diets

Vegan diets are connected to an array of different fitness blessings, consisting of blessings for:

• Cancer chance: Vegans may also advantage from a 15% decrease chance of growing or death from cancer.

• Arthritis: Vegan diets appear specially powerful at decreasing signs of arthritis including pain, joint swelling and morning stiffness.

• Kidney characteristic: Diabetics who replacement meat for plant protein may also lessen their chance of bad kidney characteristic .

- Alzheimer's disorder: Observational research display that components of the vegan eating regimen may also assist lessen the chance of growing Alzheimer's disorder .

That said, hold in thoughts that maximum of the research assisting those blessings are observational. This makes it hard to decide whether or not the vegan eating regimen at once precipitated the blessings.

Randomized managed research are wished earlier than sturdy conclusions may be made.

BOTTOM LINE:

A vegan eating regimen is connected to numerous different fitness blessings. However, greater studies is wanted to decide causality.

Foods to Avoid

Vegans keep away from ingesting any animal ingredients, in addition to any ingredients containing substances derived from animals. These encompass:

• Meat and fowl: Beef, lamb, pork, veal, horse, organ meat, wild meat, chicken, turkey, goose, duck, quail, etc.

• Fish and seafood: All kinds of fish, anchovies, shrimp, squid, scallops, calamari, mussels, crab, lobster, etc.

• Dairy: Milk, yogurt, cheese, butter, cream, ice cream, etc.

• Eggs: From chickens, quails, ostriches, fish, etc.

• Bee merchandise: Honey, bee pollen, royal jelly, etc.

• Animal-primarily based totally substances: Whey, casein, lactose, egg white albumen, gelatin, cochineal or carmine, isinglass, shellac, L-cysteine, animal-derived nutrition D3 and fish-derived omega-three fatty acids.

BOTTOM LINE:

Vegans keep away from ingesting any animal flesh, animal byproducts or ingredients containing an component from animal origin.

CHAPTER THREE

Foods to Eat

Health-aware vegans replacement animal merchandise with plant-primarily based totally replacements, including:

• Tofu, tempeh and seitan: These offer a flexible protein-wealthy opportunity to meat, fish, fowl and eggs in lots of recipes.

• Legumes: Foods including beans, lentils and peas are exceptional reassets of many vitamins and useful plant compounds. Sprouting, fermenting and right cooking can growth nutrient absorption.

• Nuts and nut butters: Especially unblanched and unroasted types, which can be properly reassets of iron, fiber, magnesium, zinc, selenium and nutrition E.

• Seeds: Especially hemp, chia and flaxseeds, which include an awesome quantity of protein and useful omega-three fatty acids.

• Calcium-fortified plant milks and yogurts: These assist vegans reap their endorsed nutritional calcium intakes. Opt for types additionally fortified with nutrients B12 and D every time possible.

• Algae: Spirulina and chlorella are properly reassets of entire protein.

Other types are extraordinary reassets of iodine.

• Nutritional yeast: This is an smooth manner to growth the protein content material of vegan dishes and upload an thrilling tacky flavor. Pick nutrition B12-fortified types every time possible.

• Whole grains, cereals and pseudocereals: These are a extraordinary supply of complicated carbs, fiber, iron, B-nutrients and numerous minerals. Spelt, teff, amaranth and quinoa are particularly excessive-protein alternatives.

• Fruits and veggies: Both are extraordinary ingredients to growth your nutrient consumption. Leafy vegetables including bok choy, spinach, kale, watercress and mustard vegetables are specially excessive in iron and calcium.

BOTTOM LINE:

These minimally processed plant ingredients are extraordinary additions to any vegan fridge or pantry.

Risks and How to Minimize Them

Favoring a properly-deliberate eating regimen that limits

processed ingredients and replaces them with nutrient-wealthy ones rather is vital for everyone, now no longer handiest vegans.

That said, the ones following poorly deliberate vegan diets are specially vulnerable to positive nutrient deficiencies.

In fact, research display that vegans are at a better chance of getting insufficient blood ranges of nutrition B12, nutrition D, long-chain omega-3s, iodine, iron, calcium and zinc.

Not getting sufficient of those vitamins is worrisome for everyone, however it is able to pose a selected chance to people with expanded necessities, including youngsters or ladies who're pregnant or breastfeeding.

Your genetic make-up and the composition of your intestine micro organism may additionally have an impact on your capacity to derive the vitamins you want from a vegan eating regimen.

One manner to reduce the chance of deficiency is to restrict the quantity of processed vegan ingredients you devour and choose nutrient-wealthy plant ingredients rather.

Fortified ingredients, particularly the ones enriched with calcium, nutrition D and nutrition B12, have to additionally make a each day look to your plate.

Furthermore, vegans looking to beautify their absorption of iron and zinc have to strive fermenting, sprouting and cooking meals.

Also, the usage of iron forged pots and pans for cooking, averting tea or espresso with food and mixing iron-wealthy ingredients with a supply of nutrition C can in addition enhance iron absorption.

Moreover, the addition of seaweed or iodized salt to the eating regimen can assist vegans attain their endorsed each day consumption of iodine.

Lastly, omega-three containing ingredients, particularly the ones excessive in alpha-linolenic acid (ALA), can assist the frame produce longer-chain omega-3s including eicosapentaenoic acid (EPA) and docosahexaenoic acid (DHA).

Foods excessive in ALA encompass chia, hemp, flaxseeds, walnuts and soybeans. However, there's debate concerning whether or not this conversion is green sufficient to fulfill each day needs.

Therefore, a each day consumption of two hundred–three hundred mg of EPA and DHA from an algae oil complement can be a more secure manner to save you low ranges.

BOTTOM LINE:

Vegans can be at an expanded chance of positive nutrient deficiencies. A properly-deliberate vegan eating regimen that consists of nutrient-wealthy entire and fortified ingredients can assist offer ok nutrient ranges.

CHAPTER FOUR

Supplements to Consider

Some vegans may also locate it hard to consume sufficient of the nutrient-wealthy or fortified ingredients above to fulfill their each day necessities.

In this case, the subsequent dietary supplements may be specially useful:

• Vitamin B12: Vitamin B12 in cyanocobalamin shape is the maximum studied and appears to paintings properly for maximum human beings.

• Vitamin D: Opt for D2 or vegan D3 bureaucracy including the ones synthetic with the aid of using Nordic Naturals or Viridian.

• EPA and DHA: Sourced from algae oil.

• Iron: Should handiest be supplemented in the case of a documented deficiency. Ingesting an excessive amount of iron from dietary supplements can motive fitness headaches and save you the absorption of different vitamins.

• Iodine: Take a complement or upload half teaspoon of iodized salt on your eating regimen each day.

• Calcium: Calcium is high-quality absorbed whilst taken in doses of

500 mg or much less at a time. Taking calcium on the identical time as iron or zinc dietary supplements may also lessen their absorption.

• Zinc: Taken in zinc gluconate or zinc citrate bureaucracy. Not to be taken on the identical time as calcium dietary supplements(64).

BOTTOM LINE:

Vegans not able to fulfill their endorsed nutrient intakes thru ingredients or fortified merchandise on my own have to recollect taking dietary supplements.

A Vegan Sample Menu for One Week

To assist get you started, here's a easy plan masking a week's really well worth of vegan food:

Monday

• Breakfast: Vegan breakfast sandwich with tofu, lettuce, tomato, turmeric and a plant-milk chai latte.

• Lunch: Spiralized zucchini and quinoa salad with peanut dressing.

• Dinner: Red lentil and spinach dalover wild rice.

Tuesday

• Breakfast: Overnight oats made with fruit, fortified plant milk, chia seeds and nuts.

• Lunch: Seitan sauerkraut sandwich.

• Dinner: Pasta with a lentil bolognese sauce and a aspect salad.

Wednesday

• Breakfast: Mango and spinach smoothie made with fortified plant milk and a banana-flaxseed-walnut muffin.

• Lunch: Baked tofu sandwich with a aspect of tomato salad.

• Dinner: Vegan chili on a mattress of amaranth.

Thursday

• Breakfast: Whole-grain toast with hazelnut butter, banana and a fortified plant yogurt.

• Lunch: Tofu noodle soup with veggies.

• Dinner: Jacket candy potatoes with lettuce, corn, beans, cashews and guacamole.

Friday

• Breakfast: Vegan chickpea and onion omelet and a cappuccino made with fortified plant milk.

• Lunch: Vegan tacos with mango-pineapple salsa.

• Dinner: Tempeh stir-fry with bok choy and broccoli.

Saturday

• Breakfast: Spinach and scrambled tofu wrap and a pitcher of fortified plant milk.

• Lunch: Spiced pink lentil, tomato and kale soup with entire-grain toast and hummus.

• Dinner: Veggie sushi rolls, miso soup, edamame and wakame salad.

Sunday

• Breakfast: Chickpea pancakes, guacamole and salsa and a pitcher of fortified orange juice.

• Lunch: Tofu vegan quiche with a aspect of sautéed mustard vegetables.

• Dinner: Vegan spring rolls.

Remember to differ your reassets of protein and veggies in the course of the day, as every affords unique nutrients and minerals which might be vital on your fitness.

BOTTOM LINE:

You can consume a lot of tasty plant-primarily based totally food on a vegan eating regimen.

CHAPTER FIVE

How to Eat Vegan at Restaurants

Dining out as a vegan may be

When eating in a non-vegan establishment, strive scanning the menu on line in advance to peer what vegan alternatives they will have for you.

Sometimes, calling in advance of time lets in the chef to set up some thing particularly for you. This lets in you to reach on the eating place assured that you'll have some thing with any luck greater thrilling than a aspect salad to reserve.

When choosing a eating place at the fly, ensure to invite approximately their vegan alternatives as quickly as you step in, preferably earlier than being seated.

When in doubt, choose ethnic eating places. They generally tend to have dishes which might be obviously vegan-pleasant or may be without difficulty changed to turn out to be so. Mexican, Thai, Middle-Eastern, Ethiopian and Indian eating places have a tendency to be extraordinary alternatives.

Once in the eating place, strive figuring out the vegetarian alternatives at the menu and asking whether or not the dairy or eggs may be eliminated to make the dish vegan-pleasant.

Another smooth tip is to reserve numerous vegan appetizers or aspect dishes to make up a meal.

BOTTOM LINE:

Being properly organized lets in you to lessen pressure whilst eating out as a vegan.

Healthy Vegan Snacks

Snacks are a extraordinary manner to live energized and hold starvation at bay among food.

Some thrilling, transportable vegan alternatives encompass:

• Fresh fruit with a dollop of nut butter

• Hummus and veggies

• Nutritional yeast sprinkled on popcorn

• Roasted chickpeas

• Nut and fruit bars

• Trail blend

• Chia pudding

- Homemade muffins

- Whole-wheat pita with salsa and guacamole

- Cereal with plant milk

- Edamame

- Whole-grain crackers and cashew nut spread

- A plant-milk latte or cappuccino

- Dried seaweed snacks

Whenever making plans a vegan snack, try and choose fiber- and protein-wealthy alternatives, which could assist hold starvation away.

BOTTOM LINE:

These transportable, fiber-wealthy, protein-wealthy vegan snacks are handy alternatives to assist reduce starvation among food.

1. Can I handiest consume uncooked meals as a vegan?

Absolutely now no longer. Although a few vegans pick to do so, uncooked veganism isn't for everyone. Many vegans consume cooked meals, and there's no medical foundation with a view to consume handiest uncooked ingredients.

2. Will switching to a vegan eating regimen assist me lose weight?

A vegan eating regimen that emphasizes nutritious, entire plant ingredients and bounds processed ones may also assist you lose weight.

As cited in the weight reduction segment above, vegan diets generally tend to assist human beings consume fewer energy while not having to consciously limit their meals consumption.

That said, whilst matched for energy, vegan diets aren't any greater powerful than different diets for weight reduction.

3 What is the high-quality milk replacement?

There are many plant-primarily based totally milk options to cow's milk. Soy and hemp types include greater protein, making them greater useful to the ones seeking to hold their protein consumption excessive.

Whichever plant milk you pick, make sure it's enriched with calcium, nutrition D and, if possible, nutrition B12.

CHAPTER SIX

Vegans generally tend to consume a whole lot of soy. Is this terrible for you?

Soybeans are extraordinary reassets of plant-primarily based totally protein. They include an array of nutrients, minerals, antioxidants and useful plant compounds which might be connected to numerous fitness blessings .

However, soy may also suppress thyroid characteristic in predisposed people and motive fueloline and diarrhea in others.

It's high-quality to choose minimally processed soy meals merchandise including tofu and edamame and restrict the usage of soy-primarily based totally mock meats.

5. How can I update eggs in recipes?

Chia and flaxseeds are a extraordinary manner to update eggs in baking. To update one egg, virtually blend one tablespoon of chia or floor flaxseeds with 3 tablespoons of warm water and permit it to relaxation till it gels.

Mashed bananas also can be a extraordinary opportunity to eggs in a few cases.

Scrambled tofu is a great vegan opportunity to scrambled eggs. Tofu also can be utilized in a lot of egg-primarily based totally recipes starting from omelets to frittatas and quiches.

6. How can I ensure I get sufficient protein?

Vegans can make sure they meet their each day protein necessities with the aid of using consisting of protein-wealthy plant ingredients of their each day food.

Check out this text for a closer examine the high-quality reassets of plant protein.

7. How can I ensure I get sufficient calcium?

Calcium-wealthy ingredients encompass bok choy, kale, mustard vegetables, turnip vegetables, watercress, broccoli, chickpeas and calcium-set tofu.

Fortified plant milks and juices also are a extraordinary manner for vegans to growth their calcium consumption.

The RDA for calcium is 1,000 mg in line with day for maximum adults and will increase to 1,two hundred mg in line with day for adults over 50 years old.

Some argue that vegans may also have barely decrease each day necessities due to the shortage of meat of their diets. Not lots medical proof may be determined to assist or negate this claim.

However, cutting-edge research display that vegans ingesting much less than 525 mg of calcium every day have an expanded chance of bone fractures.

For this reason, vegans have to goal to devour 525 mg of calcium in line with day on the very least.

8 Should I take a nutrition B12 complement?

Vitamin B12 is normally determined in animal ingredients. Some plant ingredients may also include a shape of this nutrition, however there's nevertheless debate approximately whether or not this shape is energetic in humans.

Despite circulating rumors, there's no medical proof to assist unwashed produce as a dependable supply of nutrition B12.

The each day endorsed consumption is 2.four mcg in line

with day for adults, 2.6 mcg in line with day at some stage in being pregnant and 2.eight mcg in line with day whilst breastfeeding

Vitamin B12-fortified merchandise and dietary supplements are the handiest dependable styles of nutrition B12 for vegans.

Unfortunately, many vegans appear to fail to devour enough nutrition B12 to fulfill their each day necessities.

If you're not able to fulfill your each day necessities thru the usage of nutrition B12-fortified merchandise, you have to sincerely recollect taking a nutrition B12 complement.

Individuals may also pick veganism for ethical, environmental or fitness reasons.

When performed proper, the vegan eating regimen may be smooth to observe and can offer numerous fitness blessings.

As with any eating regimen, those blessings handiest seem in case you are constant and construct your eating regimen round nutrient-wealthy plant ingredients as opposed to closely processed ones.

Vegans, particularly individuals who are not able to fulfill their each day nutrient necessities thru eating regimen on my own, have to recollect dietary supplements.

THE END

9 798320 665146